Contents

Disclaimer 2

Introduction 4

Ready – Set – Go 6

Which Diet Program will Work for You? 10

Sensible Eating Habits 21

4 Easy Changes You Can Make to Help Lose Weight 27

Final Thoughts 29

About the Author 31

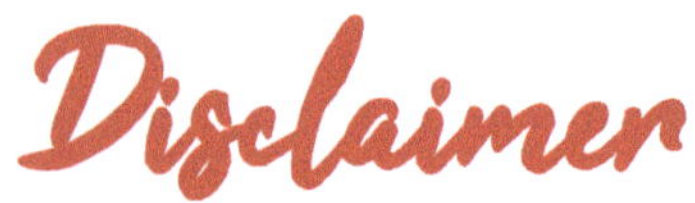

This publication is for informational purposes only and is not intended as medical advice. Medical advice should always be obtained from a qualified medical professional for any health conditions or symptoms associated with them. Every possible effort has been made in preparing and researching this material. We make no warranties with respect to the accuracy, applicability of its contents or any omissions.

See your healthcare professional before starting any diet, health or exercise program!

Published by:

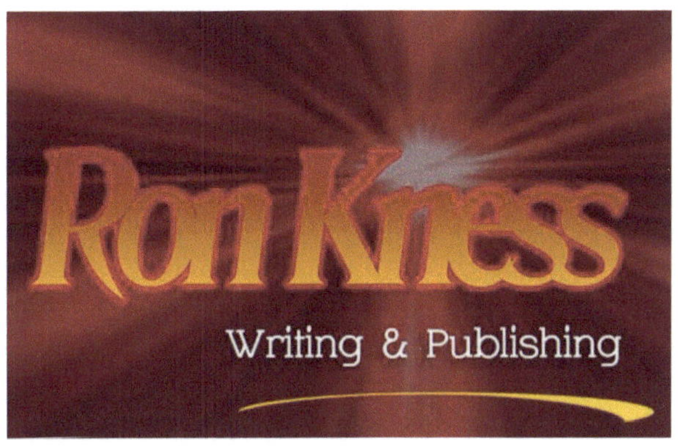

Ron Kness

San Tan Valley, AZ

United States of America

Copyright © 2019 – Ron Kness – All Rights Reserved

ISBN: 9781793051684

Introduction

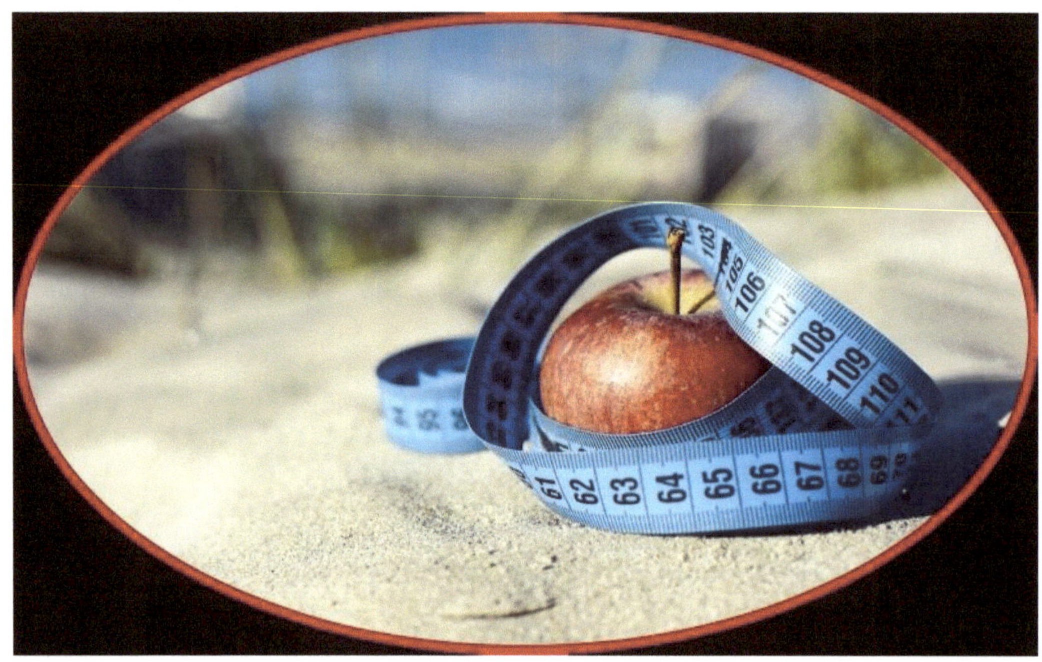

Confused about how to get started on your weight loss program? Don't know which program will work for you? Can't figure out the difference between low carb and low calorie? Or maybe you'd like to try that Paleo or Green smoothie diet everyone has been talking about. ***Blast The Fat – Lose the Weight*** answers those questions and more.

Learn which foods burn off fat; which foods have negative calories. How to avoid gaining weight when dining out. How exercise helps you boost weight loss.

Negative Calorie Foods???

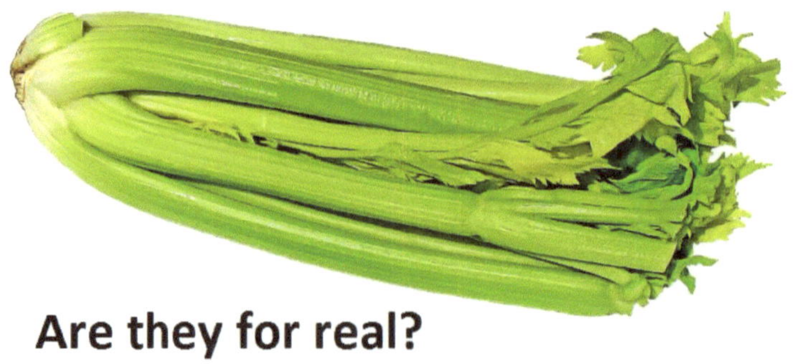

Are they for real?

But first, if you are looking for "new" and "easy" ways to lose weight, you won't find them here - they don't exist.

Losing weight is about calories – you have to burn more than you take in to lose weight. Specifically, you have to burn 3,500 more calories per week then you eat to lose one pound of weight. Eighty percent of those 3,500 calories will be from what, when and how much you eat; the other 20% will come from exercising. That is one reason why fitness experts say you can't out-exercise a bad diet. Most weight loss comes from food.

However this guide can help you make choices – choices that can help you realize your weight loss goals.

Let's get started!

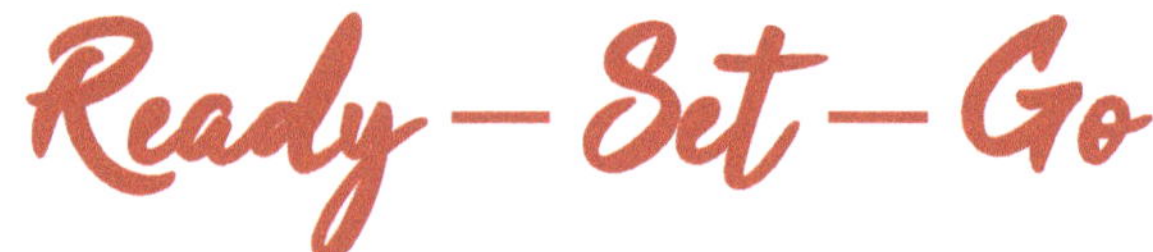

Now that you've made the choice to lose weight, prepare your mind, your environment, and your kitchen for success. Choose a day for your weight loss kick off.

Your mind is your best tool weight loss tool.

Just don't *try* to lose weight, *believe* you can lose weight. Picture yourself thin. Weight loss is as much about your **_mindset_** as it is about what you eat, when you eat and how much you eat.

Every time you weigh yourself, see your ideal weight showing up on the scale. If you have photos of yourself at your ideal weight keep them where you can glance at them often. Focus on that photo and see yourself now as you were then. Think about how comfortable your clothes will fit. How much more energy you'll have.

If it helps, think about how much more attractive your significant other will find you at your ideal weight. When you reach for a snack, tell yourself you're satisfied with what you've already eaten. Focus on the thin you inside and soon it will be a reality.

Keep a diary of the food you eat.

For the few days before you start a new eating regime, **track** exactly what you eat in a day. If you have never done this, you will be surprised! Most of us don't realize just how much food we eat in a day. We have a tendency to 'forget' the extra cream cheese with the bagel, bag of chips with lunch, mid-afternoon frozen yogurt break and bedtime snack of chocolate cookies.

Being aware of how much and what you eat is the first step to making healthful changes. If you hit a diet plateau, get out your food diary again and start keeping track. The knowledge that you will be writing down every mouthful will motivate you to stick with your routine.

A food diary serves another purpose as well. If you make a note of what you're doing and how you're feeling when you're eating, or want to eat, you may realize there are certain situations that are triggers.

When you know what triggers eating, you can prepare for it, either by avoiding the situation, or if that's not possible having a healthy snack ready to munch. Sometimes just the fact you realize that a situation has the potential for diet sabotage can help you avoid the eating response.

Plan to diet.

Make sure your scale works properly. Clean out the cupboards and fridge of foods that are too tempting. Schedule your menu for the week, or at least for several days in advance. Include healthy snacks as part of your menu.

Stock up on bottled flavored waters that are low or no sodium and no calories. Make a list of what you'll need at the grocery store and shop right after you've eaten. Hungry shoppers buy more than satisfied shoppers. Stick with your list. Don't go back to the grocery store until your next set of menus are ready to go.

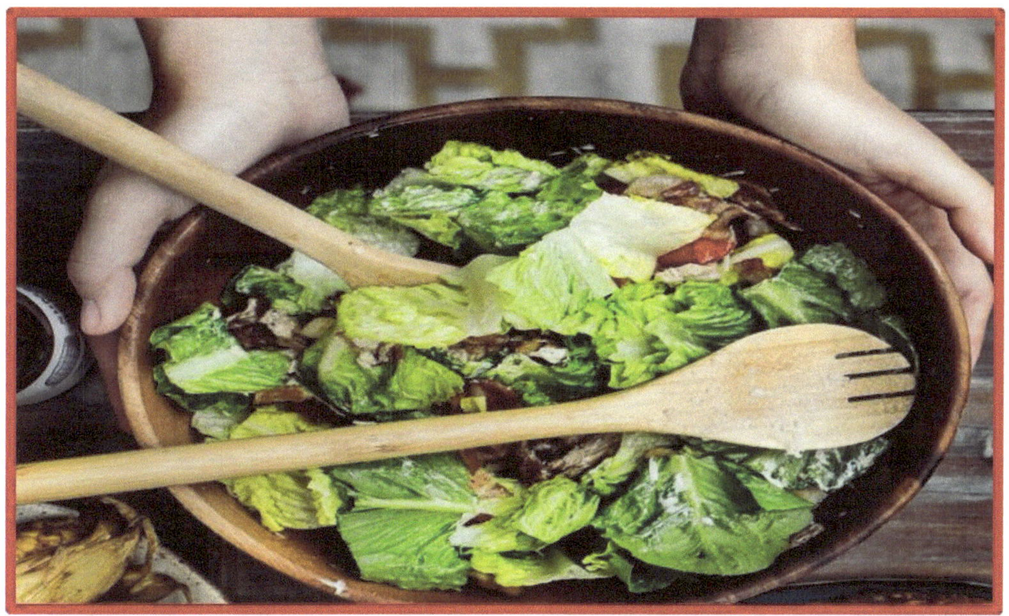

Set a goal for your weight loss and interim targets. Be realistic. If you want to lose ten pounds, it will probably take you at least two months if not more. Plan to lose at the most two pounds every week. If you're a little short one week, you can add more **exercise** or cut back on calories a bit the next week.

Stock up on fruits and veggies and prepare them in advance. Clean, peel and chop, and stash in zip lock bags so you can just grab and go. If you have to eat out, plan in advance what you will order. No bread or butter; stick with steamed vegetables, salad with dressing on the side, and broiled chicken or fish. If you just have to have that yummy sauce, ask for it on the side. You'll eat less.

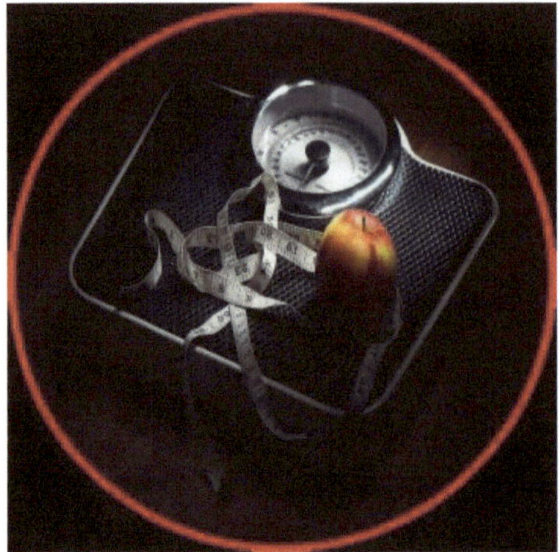

Consider enlisting your family in your weight loss program. Most of us are a bit overweight. If you need to lose a few pounds, the odds are so does your significant other. Dieting together can be more successful than dieting alone, but don't turn it into a competition.

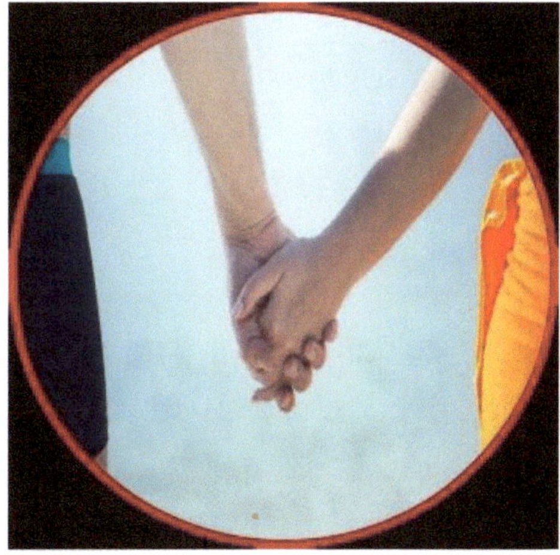

If others in your family are at their perfect weight or just don't see the need to lose weight, they may not understand the need for less food, less fat, or streamlined meals. Prepare your meal and add an extra dish or two for them that you don't particularly care for. Another alternative is to prepare your regular meal and you eat half of what you usually would eat.

Snacks and junk food can be a dieter's downfall. Buy your family their favorites that they can't live without snacks. Keep those snacks in their rooms, laundry room, or their closets. Out of your sight is out of your mouth.

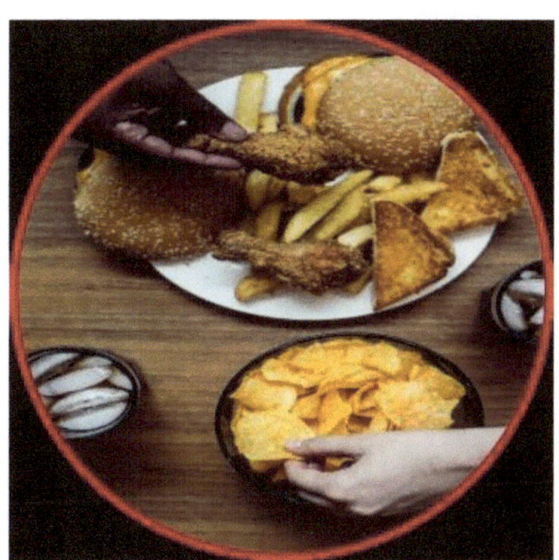

Which Diet Program will Work for You?

Low Carb

Several diet programs work on the premise that if you severely cut back carbohydrates from your diet, your body will be forced to use fat stores instead.

Carbs, especially refined carbs like sugar and flour, spike blood sugar. This spike signals the body to produce a spike of insulin in return. Insulin transfers the sugar to the body as energy. If the body doesn't need the energy at the moment it is stored as fat. Since the insulin has gotten rid of the sugar, the lack of sugar in the blood stream signals the brain it's required and you're hungry. It's a nasty cycle.

Protein, fats, and some natural carbohydrates found in vegetables, don't spike blood sugar, so the vicious cycle isn't started. Maintaining an even blood sugar level makes it easier to lose weight.

South Beach Diet and Atkins are two of the most well-known of these low carb programs.

Both start off with a two-week kickoff period that consists of eating mostly proteins supplemented by no more than 20 grams of carbs a day. A banana has 26 carbs, a slice of white bread 15, chicken 0, fats and oils 0.

Fruit, sweets, breads, and quite a few vegetables are not allowed on <u>low carb </u>programs.

After the initial kickoff, the dieter can slowly add back carbs focusing on those that don't spike your blood sugar.

The program is life long and encourages you to limit carbs, especially sugar and flour, for life.

The advantages of the low carb program are that there are few limits to the amount of low carb foods you can eat. Theoretically as much chicken, fish, beef, and cheese is allowed. Most people don't get hungry on a low carb program.

One disadvantage is that variety is restricted, so you may not get hungry but you might get bored. There may be a tendency for some people to increase their cholesterol levels while on the program if they consume too much fat or oils.

Blast the Fat – Lose the Weight

Another disadvantage is the program must be followed strictly. If you do go off the program for a special occasion, it takes several days for your body to get back to the fat burning stage.

Five hundred calories would have to be cut from the average person's daily diet to lose one pound of fat per week, that's a 20% reduction in the amount of food consumed for the average person. A restricted low-calorie program is usually between 1200 to 1500 calories per day.

A medium apple has 70 calories, an 8 oz. steak about 425. One tablespoon of fat, oil, or butter has 120 calories. As a general rule, fat and oil have more calories than any other type of food. Vegetables and fruits have the least number of calories.

Increasing the amount of exercise per day can result in weight loss. If you walk for 30 minutes daily, you'll burn off 250 calories.

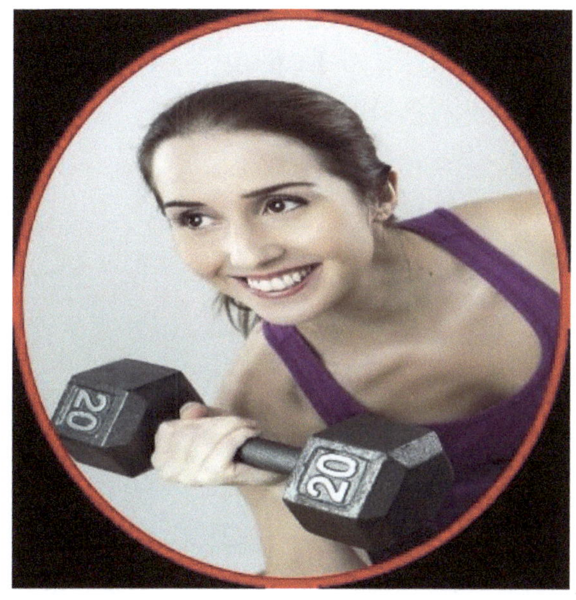

The good news is that exercising at a brisk pace, say walking, for 20 minutes will increase your metabolism from 10 to 15% for 2 to 4 hours afterward. A brisk pace means that you can still talk while walking. If you can whistle or sing, you're going too slow and if you can't catch your breath enough to hold up your end of the conversation, you're going too fast.

Combining a low-calorie program with an exercise program will allow you to burn off the fat faster.

Blast the Fat – Lose the Weight

The advantage of a low-calorie program is that you can eat a wide variety of food. There are no restrictions on what you can eat, just how much you can eat.

Low Calorie

The average person needs to eat about 2000 calories per day to maintain their weight. Of course, this varies based on how much the person weighs, their metabolism and activity levels, but it is a bench mark. There are two ways to lose weight on a low-calorie program, either cut back the number of calories consumed or increase activity levels to burn off more calories.

A pound of fat requires 3500 calories either be burned or not consumed. A calorie is the amount of energy in food.

If you absolutely must have a piece of cheesecake, you can eat it as long as you include it in your daily calorie consumption.

The disadvantages include sometimes being hungry.

Severely cutting back calories doesn't accelerate weight loss, in fact it has the opposite effect. Your body is conditioned to react to starvation, which is what you're doing when you decrease calories below 1000 per day, by lowering your metabolism. So you can cut back and your body will just compensate.

The bad news is if you go back to a normal diet it takes your body a while to realize you're not starving and increase your metabolism back to normal levels.

Prepackaged Food Programs

You've probably heard of most of them like *Jenny Craig*. You receive prepackaged foods for breakfast, lunch and dinner. Some programs also include snacks. You may add fresh diary and produce. The meals are balanced to provide all the nutrients you need and are low fat and low calorie, so you lose weight.

A variation of the prepackaged food program are the meal replacement programs. You consume a prepared drink or snack bar to replace breakfast and lunch and consume a normal low fat, or sensible dinner.

The advantage of the prepackaged food programs is that you don't have to think. You know what you can have. There are no decisions to be made. No carb counting. No calorie counting. The products have simplified diet programs.

The disadvantages include the expense of the program. The prepackaged meals are not cheap. Another disadvantage, at least in the beginning, is the shock of the small portions. Some participants recommended adding additional steamed veggies to bulk up the menu.

The bad news is if you go back to a normal diet it takes your body a while to realize you're not starving and increase your metabolism back to normal levels.

South Beach Diet: Is It the Diet For You

The South Beach Diet is similar to the Atkins Diet in that it has an initial two-week phase I period that drastically reduces carbs. The difference between Atkins and South Beach is that there are **good carbs and bad carbs**. The glycemic index of a food is what counts. The **glycemic index** is how much a food increases blood sugar compared to the amount that same quantity of white bread would increase blood sugar.

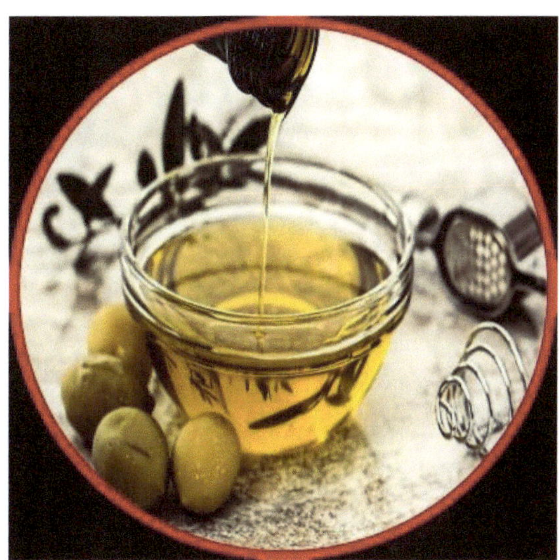

A spike in blood sugar or glucose, signals the pancreas to make more insulin. The insulin's job is to get the sugar out of the blood stream into the organs for energy or into storage. The body stores glucose as fat. Keeping the blood sugar from spiking means less insulin is produced which means the sugars are absorbed slowly resulting in a steady level of decreasing sugar levels rather than a rush. Low blood sugar leads to cravings for sugary foods and over eating. And the cycle starts again.

Bad carbs spike the blood sugar. Good carbs don't. Good carbs are those from foods which contain a lot of fiber, such as whole grains or contain fiber and water such as fruit. The body takes longer to digest the good carbs, so they enter the blood stream more slowly.

The longer food takes to digest, the better. For example, a piece of raw broccoli is better than cooked because your body must work harder to digest the raw broccoli. The faster carbohydrates are digested, the more quickly they're turned into sugar – glucose, and the more likely they will be turned to stored fat.

Fiber, protein and fats slow down the digestive system which means the blood sugar rises slowly and falls slowly. The tendency to over eat is diminished and the onset of hunger delayed.

The South Beach Diet limits fats and oils and encourages the consumption of lean cuts of meat and low-fat cheeses. Vegetables and fruits are allowed after the initial phase I - two-week period.

Whole grains can be added back including whole grain bread. White breads, cookies, cakes, rice, potatoes, and sugar are off limits except for special occasions.

 The South Beach Diet is a change in eating patterns for life, but other than the forbidden processed foods, white flour, and sugar, the diet is reasonably manageable.

It allows a broader selection of foods than the Atkins diet.

Paleo Diet

Go back to being a caveman or woman by eating only those foods that Neolithic man would eat. That means lots of meat, vegetables, and fruit but no grains, sugars, flour or processed foods.

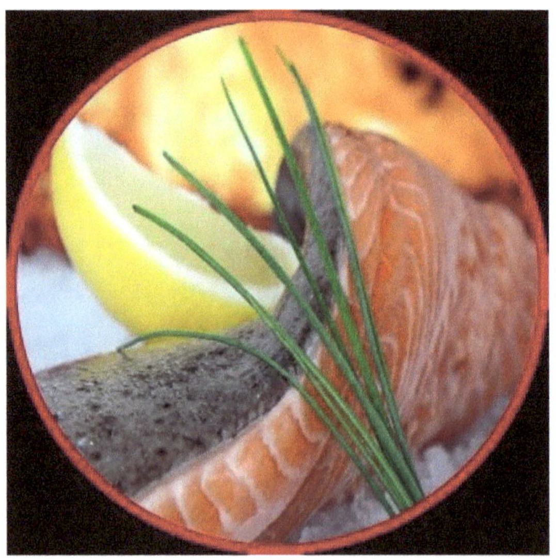

The ***Paleo Diet*** isn't as restrictive as say the low carb. For example, you could go out to eat at a fine restaurant and feast on steak, shrimp, fresh asparagus with a splash of lemon juice and fruit for dessert.

The idea behind the Paleo Diet is the human body hasn't adapted to modern convenience food and not only has trouble digesting those foods but stores them as fat.

Blast the Fat – Lose the Weight

Natural fats are allowed as is meat, poultry, fish. Calorie counting, and portion control are not encouraged. Lots of fresh and frozen vegetables, but not canned because of the high salt levels. Fruit and nuts in moderation.

The Paleo Diet isn't as restrictive as say the low carb. For example, you could go out to eat at a fine restaurant and feast on steak, shrimp, fresh asparagus with a splash of lemon juice and fruit for dessert.

What's not allowed are grains, cereals, legumes, flour and sugar, cheese or any dairy. Eggs are on the fence, since prehistoric woman probably snagged eggs from nests.

Sometimes butter is allowed as are oils from olives, coconut, and nuts. Corn, sunflower, safflower oils are not allowed.   Whether this makes sense or not doesn't matter, it's just the way of the Paleo Diet.

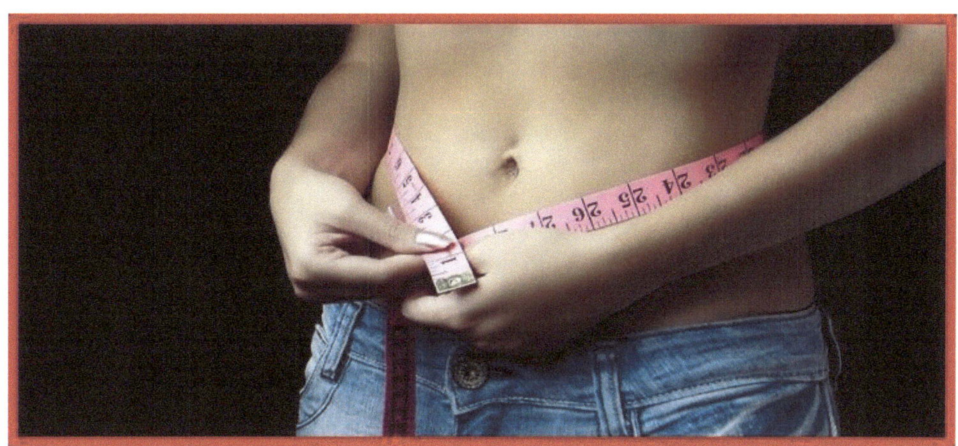

Juice Fast

Any time you drastically cut what you consume, you will lose weight. The juice fast lets you have as much freshly squeezed juices as you like. The majority of the juices must be from green vegetables with a moderate amount from sweet vegetables such as carrots and beets.

A small amount may be from fruits such as apples or berries rich in antioxidants. One juice drink a day is from nut milks to provide some protein. Herbal teas are allowed.

The juice fast is limited both in what you consume and how long you can stay on it. Fasts range from three days to three weeks.

Your body loses weight because you're drastically cutting calories and salt. However, for the long term your body adjusts its metabolism on a starvation diet to use less calories. The juice is ideal for jump starting a weight loss program.

Smoothie Diet

A take on the juice fast diet, the smoothie diet goes a step farther and adds almond milk, protein powder or whey, and yogurt to a green smoothie. The green is made from green vegetables with the addition of a small amount of fruit for sweetness. The vegetables are not juiced but blended so you do get the fiber.

Some of the smoothie recipes insist that the ingredients and portions must be followed exactly for the diet to work. Others are more lenient and allow for some creativity.

The challenge with the smoothie diet, like the juice fast, is if you don't care for raw green vegetables such as kale, spinach, or broccoli, it's difficult to stick with it. It is very limited in the variety of foods you consume.

Five Off Two On

One of the newer weight loss programs this Five Off Two On diet means you eat a sensible diet on five days but severely restrict your calories to 500 per day if you're female and 750 per day if you're male for the other two days.

Five Hundred calories isn't much. For example, a 4 oz. chicken breast is 140 calories, 55 calories in one cup of cooked broccoli, 95 calories in one medium apple. One egg is 78 calories, 90 calories in a cup of milk, 80 in one slice of bread. The two days on don't have to be consecutive.

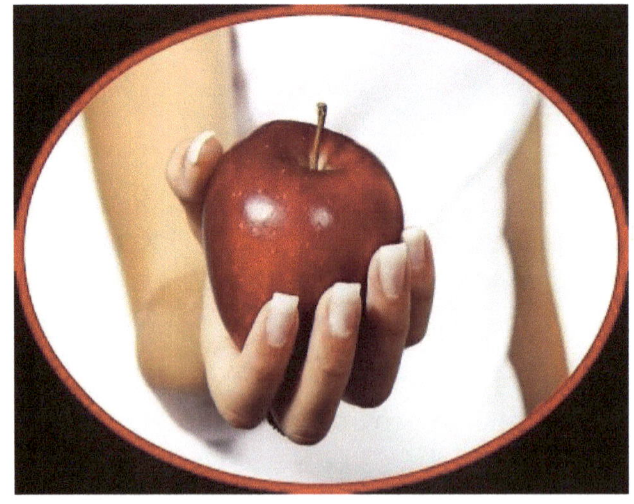

Three Day Diet

Blast the Fat – Lose the Weight

The 3 Day Diet depends on severely restricting calories for 3 days. It's not dependent on a special combination of foods. Depending on how heavy you are to start with you could lose up to 10 pounds in those three days. Keep in mind that if you weight close to 250 pounds you'll lose more than someone who weighs 150 pounds.

Some of that weight will be water because as you restrict calories you're also restricting the amount of salt you're consuming. Less salt means you'll retain less water.

Below is an example of a 3-Day Diet:

- Breakfast:
    - 1/2 grapefruit or juice; 1 slice toast with 1T of peanut butter or cottage cheese
    - 1 egg (any style); 1 slice toast; 1 banana, or
    - 5 saltine crackers; 1 slice cheddar cheese; 1 apple, or
    - 1 hard boiled egg; 1 slice toast;
- Lunch:
    - 1/2 cup tuna; 1 slice toast, or
    - 1 cup cottage cheese or tuna; 5 saltine crackers; or
    - 1 hard boiled egg; 1 slice toast
- Dinner:
    - 3 oz. any lean meat; 1 cup green beans; 1 cup carrots; 1 cup vanilla ice cream; or
    - 2 beef franks or hot dogs; 1/2 cup carrots; 1 banana; 1 cup broccoli or cabbage; 1/2 cup vanilla ice cream, or
    - 1 cup tuna; 1 cup carrots; 1 cup cauliflower; 1 cup melon; 1/2 cup vanilla ice

On this diet, you can drink as much ***black coffee***, tea or water as you like. Also, use whatever spices you like. Use cooking spray. For snacks cucumbers, celery, radishes and leafy greens are fine with a squirt of lemon juice if you like.

The challenge with this diet is that you aren't developing new eating habits. When you stop the diet you go back to your old habits and the weight returns. However, if you use this diet as a jumpstart to a healthy eating program, the weight will stay off.

ABS The ABC's of Diets

David Zinczenko is the author of "ABS The ABCs of Diets" and is the editor-in-chief of Men's Health Magazine. This diet is based on 12 power foods and a healthy eating plan.

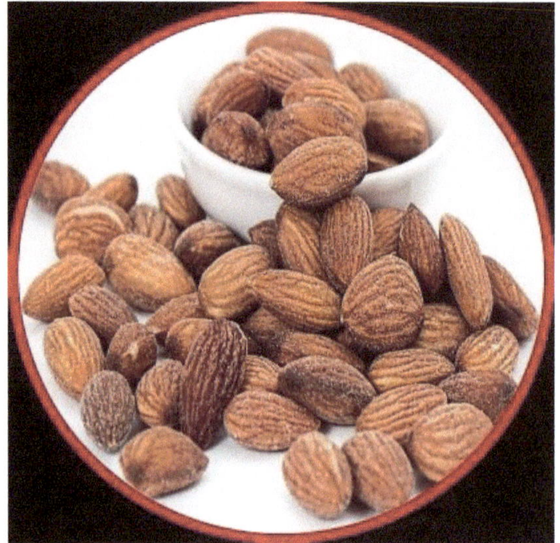

1. Almonds and other nuts

2. Beans and other legumes

3. Spinach and other green veggies

4. Dairy (fat-free/low fat)

5. Instant Oatmeal

6. Eggs

7. Turkey/lean meat

8. Peanut butter (all natural; limit to 3T per day max)

9. Olive Oil (Extra Virgin)

10. Whole grain bread/cereal

11. Extra (whey) protein powder

12. Raspberries and other berries

In case you haven't noticed the first letter of each of these foods spells "ABS DIET POWER."

That might help you remember the 12 foods.

Blast the Fat – Lose the Weight

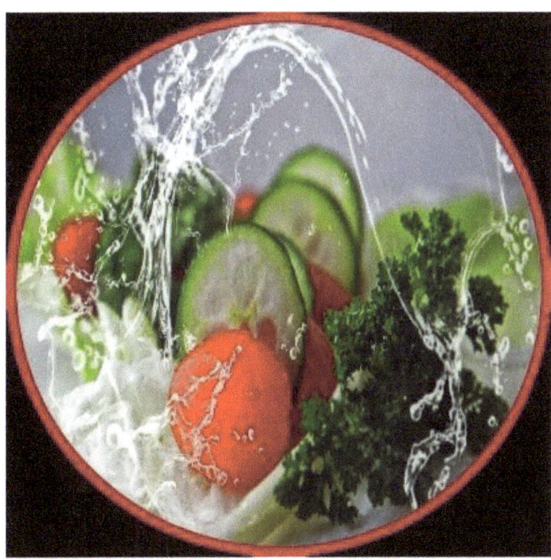

The ABS diet includes lists of other foods that can be consumed as often as you like, only occasionally, or are forbidden. For example, vegetables, fruits and lean meats are included as often as you like or occasionally while sugars are on the do not consume list

Claims for the diet include fast weight loss primarily from stomach fat first. If you want to increase muscle mass there is an exercise component to the diet -- six pack abs here you come.

ABS is a healthy eating program. However, it is restrictive because of the foods on the no list. If you can get past that, you shouldn't have a problem following the diet to not only lose weight but as a lifetime eating program.

An added plus is that vegetarians can follow the diet with a few adjustments. However, vegans -- those who consume no animal products or made by animals products -- think eggs and dairy - won't be able to follow the ABS program.

If you are the type of person who needs a program and specific plan to follow this is the eating program for you. Follow the rules, including portion size and you will lose weight.

Best Life Diet

Bob Green, Oprah's personal trainer created The Best Life Diet, which is endorsed by Oprah. The diet is popular because of Oprah's popularity on the one hand. On the other hand Oprah's weight has fluctuating over the years so it's obvious she doesn't always stick to it.

A serious challenge to anyone trying to lose weight is breaking bad eating habits. It takes 21 days to change an old habit. Quite a few people eat, not because they're hungry but for emotional reasons -- boredom, joy, depression, worry, anxiety ... the list goes on. And it's these times that junk food is the most tempting. There's no muss or fuss, just a trip to the vending machine.

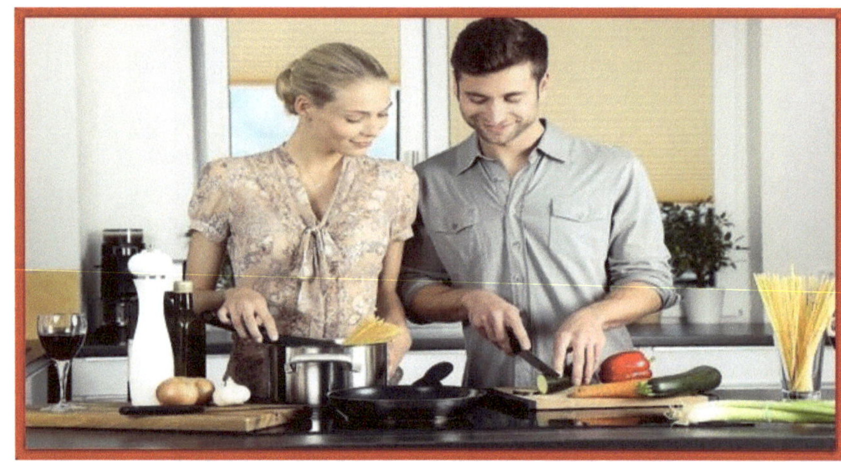

The Best Life Diet tackles emotional eating. It **_retrains your mind_** and your body to eat only when hungry and to make good healthy choices when you do eat. Combine the **_diet program with an exercise program_** and you are well on your way to a healthier thinner you.

The Best Life Diet doesn't restrict or eliminate any foods. Sometimes a dieter's downfall is wanting to eat food that is forbidden.

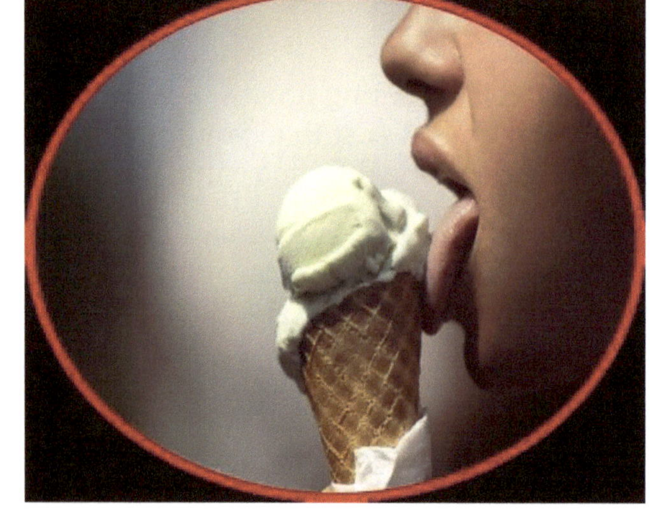

They substitute in another food that isn't satisfying but eat more of it and still aren't satisfied. So have your 1/2 cup of ice cream, savor it and then pick healthy choices for the rest of the day.

The Best Life Diet isn't really a diet for a limited time for weight loss but a healthy eating program for the rest of your life. It definitely is a **_lifestyle change_**, not just a temporary change until that excess weight is gone.

Sensible Eating Habits

Ketogenic Diet

The ___ketogenic diet___ is similar to the low carb diet but with a difference in that it's high in fat as well as low in carbohydrates. The theory is to change the body from burning sugar for fuel into burning fat for fuel. When that happens the fat stores go through the liver and are changed to fatty acids and ketones. The ketones provide the energy for the body.

The ideal ketogenic diet relies on fats for 70% of the food, 25% protein and carbs 5%. For a 2000 calorie diet that means only 100 calories from carbs or about one medium size apple.

A sample dinner could be a chicken breast sautéed in olive oil with broccoli smothered in cheese. Adding fat to nearly every meal is essential to achieving 70% fat.

As you can see the diet is very restrictive. Eating out is not a viable option since while you might think a fast food hamburger sans bun would be okay, it may not be. That burger can't have mustard, mayo, or ketchup. There can be no fillers in the hamburger which contain carbs.

The downside to the diet is that it takes the body up to 48 hours to achieve the state of ketosis once carbs have been severely limited. So if you slip up and have too many carb its takes that same amount to get back to ketosis.

Clean Eating

More of an eating program rather than a diet, ___clean eating___ focuses on consuming unprocessed, preferably organic foods in moderate quantities. Veggies, fruits, legumes, grains, and healthy low-fat proteins, such as chicken, are the backbone of clean eating programs.

The emphasis is on cooking or preparing ingredients yourself without the additives and preservatives found in say, a frozen entrée. Red meat is limited as are full-fat diary products.

Oils and other fats are limited as well. Avoid white flour, refined sugar, pastas, breads, cakes, cookies and so forth.

What you drink counts in your calories for the day.

It's easy to forget that fruit juice, sodas, sweetened ice tea, and café mocha, all add up. Water is always your best bet as a refreshing drink. Add a ***slice of lemon or lime*** for flavor. Or a crushed strawberry, a few raspberries or a peach slice. Keep a pitcher of ice water on your desk, or kitchen counter and it will remind you to drink more.

Keep single serving bottles in the freezer to grab on your way out. Put the bottled water in front of the juice, milk, and sodas and you'll be tempted to drink the water instead of the other liquids. Just cutting out two sodas a day can significantly drop your calorie count.

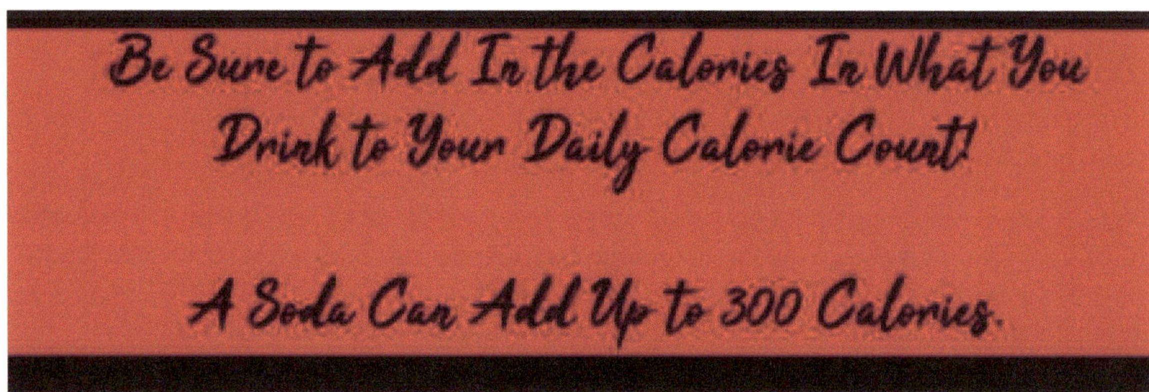

Always put food on a plate.

Use a real plate, not a paper plate, and eat at the table. You'll be amazed at how much food you consume away from meal times or on the run. It's easy to down a bag of potato chips eating in front of the TV. Or you're hungry so you grab a leftover chicken leg and eat it over the sink. You're late for work so you reach for a donut to have with your latte as you drive.

Don't eat unless you're sitting down at the table with a plate in front of you. You'll feel silly putting chips and dip on a lunch plate, so silly you probably won't do it. Putting all the food on plates and eating at the table makes you aware of how much you're eating and when – called mindful eating verses the other way discussed which is mindless eating. Seeing all the dirty plates in the sink can motivate you not to eat.

Sugar free and low fat doesn't necessarily mean low calorie.

Many of the sugar free snacks contain as many, if not more, calories than their counterparts. Low fat might mean sugar and starches have been added to make up for the lost flavor and creaminess from the fat.

Read the labels to make sure you're getting what you think you're getting. Sometimes it's better to use a lesser amount of the original food than the usual amount of the low fat or sugar-free substitute.

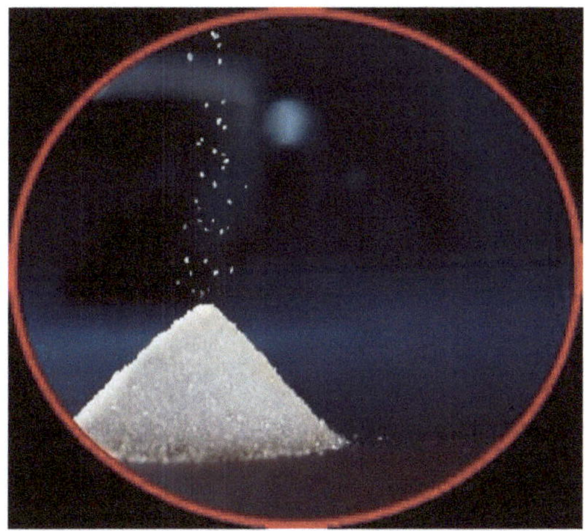

Have a fruit, or vegetable, appetizer before lunch and dinner.

We all need more fruits and vegetables in our diet. A recent study showed that most adults don't get anywhere near the recommended 5 servings a day. Fruits and vegetables are filling, low in calories and high in vitamins, minerals and enzymes. It takes about 20 minutes for your brain to get the signal from your stomach that you're full.

If you start with an appetizer you've got a head start on the clock. By the time you get to dessert, you'll feel satisfied.

Blast the Fat – Lose the Weight

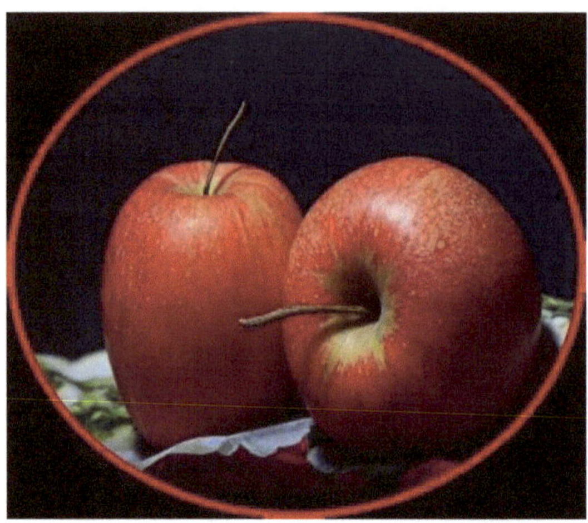

Portion Control

Know what a serving really is. Portions these days have become gigantic. You might think that a serving of cooked pasta is a big bowl full but look on the package.

You'll be surprised to see that a serving is considered just an 8-ounce cupful of cooked pasta. And the serving of pasta sauce?

Well that's just ¼ cup or 2 ounces. A serving of chicken, or meat, is 4 ounces, that's a chicken thigh or drumstick. In the case of meat, a serving is about the size of a deck of playing cards.

A serving of vegetables is ½ cup, a serving of fruit is ½ cup, or one whole fruit such as an apple. Of course, with fruits and vegetables you can be very generous with the servings. And with meat, be stingy.

Adjust your plate size. The tendency is to fill our plates full, so trick yourself and use a smaller plate. Use a 9" salad plate instead of your normal 12" dinner plate and you'll automatically eat less.

Use a small bowl instead of a soup bowl and you'll cut calories. You can also reverse it. Use the dinner plate and fill it full of salad greens – just be careful with the salad dressing. To cut down on the amount of dressing consumed, place the dressing in a small bowl on the side.

Then dip your fork in the dressing before you spear your salad. While your salad is on the dinner plate, use the salad plate for your entrée.

Use the 50-25-25 rule. 50% of what you eat should be vegetables and fruits. 25% should be grains and cereals and 25% should be protein.

Fruit, sweets, breads, and quite a few vegetables are not allowed on low carb programs.

After the initial kickoff the dieter can slowly add back carbs focusing on those that don't spike your blood sugar.

The program is life long and encourages you to limit carbs, especially sugar and flour for life.

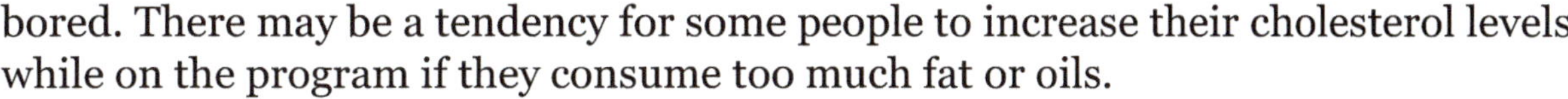

The advantages of the low carb program are that there are few limits to the amount of low carb foods you can eat. Theoretically as much chicken, fish, beef, and cheese is allowed. Most people don't get hungry on a low carb program.

One disadvantage is that variety is restricted, so you may not get hungry but you might get bored. There may be a tendency for some people to increase their cholesterol levels while on the program if they consume too much fat or oils.

Another disadvantage is the program must be followed strictly. If you do go off the program for a special occasion, it takes several days for your body to get back to the fat burning stage.

Depend on flavor not fat.

Fat tastes good. It adds satisfying creaminess and richness to foods. Cutting down on fat, including butter, oils, salad dressing and mayonnaise leads to a thinner you. Substitute herbs and spices to foods and you won't miss the fat as much.

For example, in your salad add a handful of herbs like basil with a tablespoon of parmesan cheese and a squeeze of lemon and you might not even miss the salad dressing.

In the world of weight loss, there really isn't anything new. It still comes down to burning more calories than you take in. However, here are 4 easy changes that you might not have thought of or did know at one time but have forgotten. Try them – they can make a big difference in your weight loss efforts.

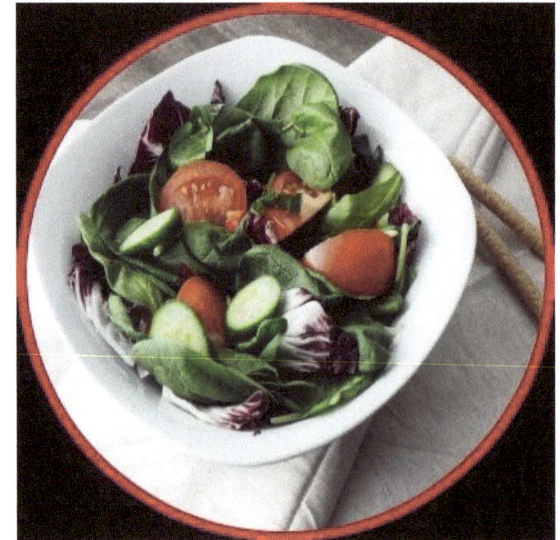

4 Easy Changes You Can Make to Help Lose Weight

Are You Really Hungry?

Are you really hungry? Or are you thirsty, bored or stressed? Often we reach for food when what we really want is to relax, have something to drink, or be entertained. Think about why you want to eat before you down that cookie. Instead of eating, have a drink of water, then wait 10 or 15 minutes.

Often the urge to eat will disappear. You can also try changing your environment to snap out of boredom. If you're sitting on the couch reading, get up and take a brief walk. Deep breathing, listening to soothing music, or taking a warm bath can bring down stress levels.

Drink Green Tea

Green tea can boost your metabolism which means you'll lose weight faster. Brew a pot of tea in the morning and keep it hot for most of the day in a thermos. Or you can ice it, add a few slices of lemon and lime and you'll have a refreshing summer drink.

The taste of green tea doesn't appeal to everyone. You can take capsules of green tea extract. You can add a flavoring to the tea. Or you can brew your tea with a ratio of one bag of green tea to one bag of black tea.

Cut the Salt

Excess salt in your diet leads to water retention and bloat. Salt is vital to a healthy body but most of us ingest way too much of it. It's hidden everywhere in processed foods such as frozen dinners and canned soups. Many restaurants use salt as the primary flavoring ingredient.

If you're used to salting everything it will be a challenge to use less. Food will taste bland for the first day or so. The best way is to go cold turkey. Don't salt anything for 72 hours and don't use any prepared foods that include salt as an ingredient.

Check the labels, you'll be surprised at where you'll find salt hiding. After the 72 hours you'll most likely find that you don't want nearly the <u>salt</u> you used to.

Use the Barter System

There are times when you want a forbidden food so much it's almost painful. Decide in advance an exercise you will do for a certain length of time in exchange for allowing yourself the forbidden food. It could be walking for 30 minutes, 100 tummy crunches, or riding a stationary bike for 15 minutes.

When you have just got to have that cappuccino mocha, do the exchange <u>first</u> before you have the mocha. Don't' say 'well I'll have mocha and when I get home tonight I'll walk for 30 minutes,' that doesn't work.

The trick is that you must do the exercise first. A lot of time it's just not convenient to exercise. For example: you might be at the office. Exercising works to decrease your appetite so when you finish you might not even want that mocha. And if you do have the mocha, you've worked off a lot of the calories with the exercise.

Final Thoughts

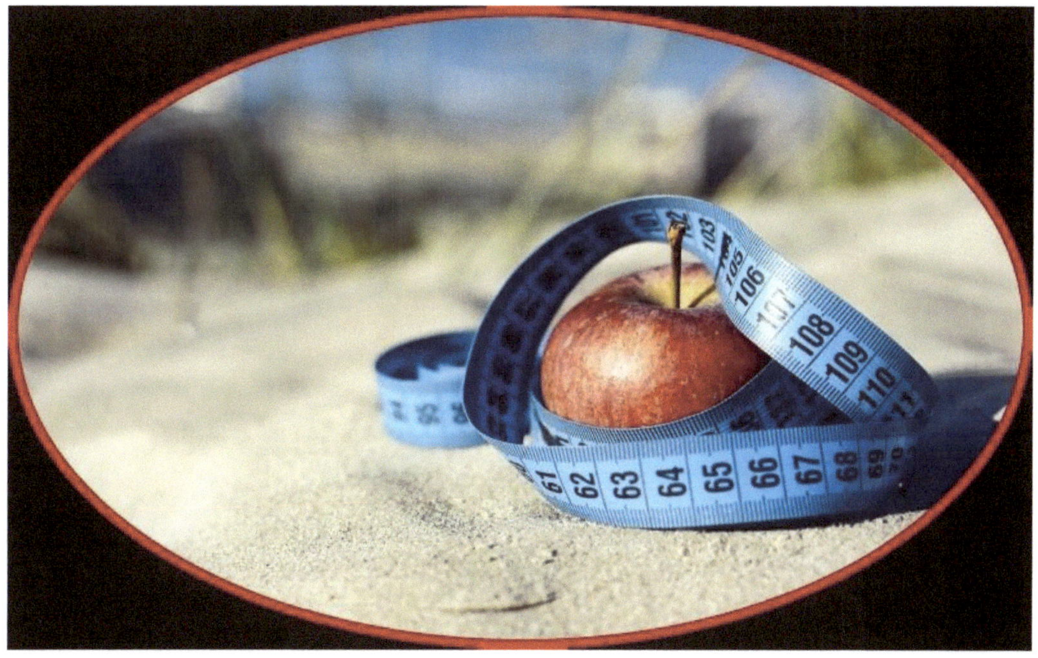

Losing weight is all about making choices – wise, healthy choices. In this guide we discussed several different diet programs that you can try to see if they in fact work for you. Sometimes it takes some experimentation before you find one right for you.

Keep in mind that most "diet" programs are meant for the short-term – to take off a few pounds quickly. Most of them are not designed for the long term.

After taking off a ***few quick pounds***, switch to a healthy ***eating*** and ***exercising*** lifestyle, so that you don't put the weight back on again. Choose a comprehensive program that you can live with for life.

While reading through this guide you may have noticed some words underlined. These are links that when clicked will take you to other publications on that topic that may be of interest to you.

As mentioned early in the guide, there isn't a new or easy way to lose weight – it takes hard work, consistency and dedication. If you have tried to lose weight before and failed, give it one more try using the information in this guide and ancillary information in the links.

You can do this!

12-Diet Rotation Plan: Try Each of These 12 Plans to See Which One Works Best for You!

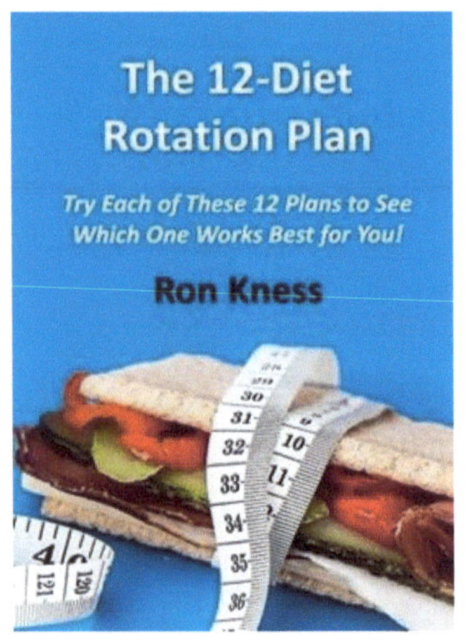

The 12-Diet Rotation Plan book provides an overview and instructions on how to use twelve of the most popular types of diets in use today:

1. 3-Hour Metabolism
2. Blood Sugar
3. Calorie Control
4. Fasting
5. Low Carb
6. Low Fat
7. Meal Replacement
8. Meatless
9. Mediterranean
10. Mindful Eating
11. Paleo
12. Sugar Detox

In each diet, you will find the following information:

•Basic principles of a that diet

•Who that diet best works for

•How to get prepared for that diet

•Sample meal plan for that specific diet

•Tips to increase success

The theory behind the plan is that the reader can rotate through each type of diet for two weeks to a month and through the recording of results, see which diet(s) has the most success for that person.

Get your copy at: https://www.amazon.com/gp/product/1981113878

About the Author

I grew up in Central Minnesota, where my parents owned and operated a fishing resort. Once out of high school I tried a couple of semesters of college, only to quit halfway through the Spring term; I decided at that time that college wasn't for me.

Then I decided to follow my father's previous occupation as an auto mechanic. I graduated from a two-year of vocational training course and worked as a mechanic for five years. While in vocational training, I decided to join the National Guard where I eventually ended up working full-time for 32 years.

So how does all of this relate to writing? In one of my leadership schools, the instructor, who was an English teacher at a juvenile detention center, presented writing to me in a whole new way - a way that started to develop my interest in working with words.

I eventually went back to college on the GI Bill taking a class or two per semester at night and on weekends took me seven years to complete my degree.

Fast forward about 40 years and now besides my own writing, I also ghostwrite ebooks, reports, articles, blogs and do Kindle conversions for clients on a variety of topics.

Today my wife and I are retired from our careers and live in Gold Canyon, AZ where you'll find me happily sitting in my office typing away as I work on my next book or ghostwriting project . . . that is if we are not traveling on a cruise ship - our new-found mode of travel.